THE ONLY INTERMITTENT FASTING BOOK YOU WILL EVER NEED

A STEP BY STEP PLAN

OVERVIEW

Intermittent Fasting (IF) refers to dietary eating patterns that involve not eating or severely restricting calories for a prolonged period. There are many different subgroups of intermittent fasting each with individual variation in the duration of the fast; some for hours, others for a day(s). This has become an extremely popular topic in the science community due to all of the potential benefits on fitness and health that are being discovered.

WHAT IS INTERMITTENT FASTING (IF)?

Fasting or periods of voluntary abstinence from food has been practised throughout the world for ages. Intermittent fasting to improve health relatively new. Intermittent fasting involves restricting the intake of food for a set period and does not include any changes to the actual foods you are eating. Currently, the most common IF protocols are a daily 16 hour fast and fasting for a whole day, one or two days per week. Intermittent fasting could be considered a natural eating pattern that humans are built to implement and it traces back to our palaeolithic hunter-gatherer ancestors. The current model of a planned program of intermittent fasting could potentially help improve many aspects of health from body composition to longevity and ageing. Although IF goes against the norms of our culture and common daily routine, the science may be pointing to less meal frequency and more time fasting as the optimal alternative to the normal breakfast, lunch, and dinner model. Here are two common myths that pertain to intermittent fasting. Myth 1 - You Must Eat 3 Meals Per Day: This "rule" that is common in Western society was not developed based on evidence for improved health, but was adopted as the common pattern for settlers and eventually became the norm. Not only is there a lack of scientific rationale in the 3 meal-a-day models, but recent studies may also be showing fewer meals and more fasting to be optimal for human health. One study showed that one meal a day with the same amount of daily calories is better for weight loss and body composition than 3 meals per day. This finding is a basic concept that is extrapolated into intermittent fasting and those choosing to do IF may find it best to only eat 1-2 meals per day.

Myth 2 - You Need Breakfast, It's The Most Important Meal of The Day:

Many false claims about the absolute need for a daily breakfast have been made. The most common claims being "breakfast increases your metabolism" and "breakfast decreases food intake later in the day". These claims have been refuted and studied over 16 weeks with results showing that skipping breakfast did not decrease metabolism and did not increase food intake at lunch and dinner. It is still possible to do intermittent fasting protocols while still eating breakfast, but some people find it easier to eat a late breakfast or skip it altogether and this common myth should not get in the way.

TYPES OF INTERMITTENT FASTING:

Intermittent fasting comes in various forms and each may have a specific set of unique benefits. Each form of intermittent fasting has variations in the fasting-to-eating ratio. The benefits and effectiveness of these different protocols may differ on an individual basis and it is important to determine which one is best for you. Factors that may influence which one to choose include health goals, daily schedule/routine, and current health status. The most common types of IF are alternate day fasting, time-restricted feeding, and modified fasting.

1. ALTERNATE DAY FASTING: This approach involves alternating days of absolutely no calories (from food or beverage) with days of free feeding and eating whatever you want. This plan has been shown to help with weight loss, improve blood cholesterol and triglyceride (fat) levels, and improve markers for inflammation in the blood. The main downfall with this form of intermittent fasting is that it is the most difficult to stick with because of the reported hunger during fasting days.

2. MODIFIED FASTING - 5:2 DIET

Modified fasting is a protocol with programmed fasting days, but the fasting days do allow for some food intake. Generally 20-25% of normal calories are allowed to be consumed on fasting days; so if you normally consume 2000 calories on regular eating days, you would be allowed 400-500 calories on fasting days. The 5:2 part of this diet refers to the ratio of non-fasting to fasting days. So on this regimen, you would eat normally for 5 consecutive days, then fast or restrict calories to 20-25% for 2 consecutive days. This protocol is great for weight loss, body composition, and may also benefit the regulation of blood sugar, lipids, and inflammation. Studies have shown the 5:2 protocol to be effective for weight loss, improve/lower inflammation markers in the blood (3), and show signs of trending improvements in insulin resistance. In animal studies, this modified fasting 5:2 diet resulted in decreased fat, decreased hunger hormones (leptin), and increased levels of a protein responsible for improvements in fat burning and blood sugar regulation (adiponectin). The modified 5:2 fasting protocol is easy to follow and has a small number of negative side effects which included hunger, low energy, and some irritability when beginning the program. Contrary to this, however, studies have also noted improvements such as reduced tension, less anger, less fatigue, improvements in self-confidence, and a more positive mood.

3. TIME-RESTRICTED FEEDING: If you know anyone that has said they are doing intermittent fasting, odds are it is in the form of time-restricted feeding. This is a type of intermittent fasting that is used daily and it involves only consuming calories during a small portion of the day and fasting for the remainder. Daily fasting intervals in time-restricted feeding may range from 12-20 hours, with the most common method being 16/8 (fasting for 16 hours, consuming calories for 8). For this protocol, the time of day is not important as long as you are fasting for a consecutive period and only eating in your allowed period. For example, on a 16/8 time-restricted feeding program one person may eat their first meal at 7 AM and last meal at 3 PM (fast from 3 PM-7 AM), while another person may eat their first meal at 1 PM and last meal at 9 PM (fast from 9 PM-1 PM). This protocol is meant to be performed every day over long periods and is very flexible as long as you are staying within the fasting/eating window(s). Time-Restricted feeding is one of the easiest to follow methods of intermittent fasting. Using this along with your daily work and sleep schedule may help achieve optimal metabolic function. Time-restricted feeding is a great program to follow for weight loss and body composition improvements as well as some other overall health benefits. The few human trials that were conducted noted significant reductions in weight, reductions in fasting blood glucose, and improvements in cholesterol with no changes in perceived tension, depression, anger, fatigue, or confusion. Some other preliminary results from animal studies showed time-restricted feeding to protect against obesity, high insulin levels, fatty liver disease, and inflammation. The easy application and promising results of time-restricted feeding could make it an excellent option for weight loss and chronic disease prevention/management. When implementing this protocol it may be good, to begin with, a lower fasting-to-eating ratio like 12/12 hours and eventually work your way up to 16/8 hours.

COMMON QUESTION ABOUT INTERMITTENT FASTING:

Is there any food or beverage I am allowed to consume while intermittent fasting? Unless you are doing the modified fasting 5:2 diet (mentioned above), you should not be eating or drinking anything that contains calories. Water, black coffee, and any foods/beverages that do not contain calories are OK to consume during a fasting period. Adequate water intake is essential during IF and some say that drinking black coffee while fasting helps decrease hunger.

Intermittent fasting that is currently the most popular health and fitness method globally is also known as IF. People are using this method as a way to reduce weight, improve their overall health, and also to simplify their lifestyles. Most studies suggest that it can give powerful effects on different systems in the body and brain and let the practice live longer. Through the following guide, you will know the most basic things and concepts about intermittent fasting. What Essentially Is Intermittent Fasting? F or intermittent fasting is a certain eating pattern in cycles between fasting and eating sessions. It doesn't necessarily specify which foods you must eat in the eating cycle. Instead, it lets you know at what times you must eat. In this way, it isn't a diet in the actual meanings but is more of an eating pattern. The most common intermittent fasting includes 16 hours of fasts or having 24 hours of fast two times a week. Fasting has always been involved in the common practices of the human evolution period. Ancient hunter-gatherers never had refrigerators, supermarkets, or foods that were available to them throughout the year. And many times they couldn't find anything to eat at all. And as a result, human beings evolved to live their lives without any food for long periods. Fasting from time to time is a natural method of overeating over 3 to 4 meals in a day. Fasting is also mostly done in religious practices that include religions like Christianity, Islam, Judaism, and

Buddhism. What Are A Few Intermittent Fasting Methods? There are many different methods of practicing intermittent fasting, most of which involve breaking it the day or week into fasting and eating periods. During the sessions of fasting, you may eat a little or not even a bit. The most popular methods of intermittent fasting are as follows: The 16/8 method: This is also called the Leangains protocol that involves not having breakfast and restricting the daily eating pattern to only 8 hours, such as 1 to 9 pm. Then you should fast for 16 hours during the session. Eat stop eat: This is the process of fasting for 24 hours only once or twice a week, i.e. not eating from dinner to another dinner. And the rest of the week you spend is normal like your daily life. The 5:2 diet: This method includes consumption of only 500 to 600 calories on days that are not consecutive of a week. You normally eat for the rest of the 5 days. By reducing the total calorie intake, all these methods must cause a weight loss as long as you are not compensating by having too much to eat in the eating sessions. Many people also find out that the 16/8 method is the simplest one to follow. It is also the most sustainable and easy to stick to. Hence it is the most popular method of intermittent fasting. How Does Intermittent Fasting Affect Our Cells And Hormones? When you are fasting, many things happen to the body on a molecular and cellular level. For example, the body starts adjusting to the hormonal levels to make the stored body fat a lot more accessible. Your cells also start the important repairing process and change the expression of the genes. A few changes that happen in the body are as follows: Human growth hormone, i.e. HGH: The growth of humans, boosts to folds in intermittent fasting. This has many benefits that include a fast fat loss and a few to mention a muscle gain. Insulin: Insulin sensitivity gets a lot better, and the levels of insulin fast in intermittent fasting. The lower levels of insulin make the stored body fat be more accessible. Cellular repair: When you have fasted for a while, your cells start the cellular repair process. This also includes autophagy where these cells digest and remove the old protein that starts building up. Gene expression: There are many changes in the functioning of genres linked to the protection and longevity against a disease. Knowing that intermittent fasting helps make your body systems improve to many folds, are you ready to start doing it in your life.

BENEFITS OF INTERMITTENT FASTING.

Intermittent fasting is not so much a diet but a pattern or timing of how to eat. It is how early mankind fed itself for millennia. It has many benefits to improve our health. This article discusses intermittent fasting (IF), types of intermittent fasting and subsequent health benefits. To be very clear this article is meant for general purposes and should not be utilized individually, but in consultation with one's health care provider. Let's begin with stating that intermittent fasting means NO SNACKS! Snacking is out. Intermittent means we will wait an interval of time between meals. There are various patterns that can be used for intermittent fasting. One of the simplest is: 3 square meals a day. This is a time-honored custom for many in the boomer generation and previous generations. It involves having breakfast, lunch and dinner and not eating overnight. Typically, a 4-5 hour time span between meals occurs. Since each meal is substantial the individual doesn't become hungry. Another method of IF is to utilize the 3 square meals a day and to add a 24-48 hour fasting time once a month where one only drinks water and sparingly drinks a vegetable broth. There are a number of other patterns that can be pursued and are readily investigated by consulting an expert of nutrition and online references. The benefits of IF are numerous, ranging from weight loss, improved metabolism, decreased chronic pain and lower risk of cancer. Weight loss occurs when we refrain from eating for longer periods. If we eat frequently, we are constantly burning calories from the food we've consumed. However, by utilizing IF we burn fat and subsequently lose weight. Many people feel that their metabolism is slow or unstable. Intermittent fasting can speed up and stabilize overall body metabolism. Physiologically IF reduces the amount of insulin produced by the pancreas and allows blood glucose levels to normalize. Over weeks and months metabolic activities of the body naturally become more balanced, normal and regular. Intermittent fasting has been shown to reduce the type of white blood cell called monocytes. Monocytes are linked with body inflammation. By decreasing inflammation chronic musculoskeletal pains can be improved. Cancer cells typically feed on glucose. Blood glucose is high when we snack and eat frequently. Conversely, when we fast intermittently, we burn fat. Since most cancer cells cannot feed on fat cancer risk lessons. Some studies show that intermittent fasting helps the body to clean out toxins and damaged cells. This cleansing and purification reduces tiredness and sluggishness and helps boost energy. Fasting, in general, is an age-old process that dates back centuries to many faiths and cultures. Almost everyone can easily engage in intermittent fasting and there are a wide array of health benefits.

When it comes to weight loss and what to do to get that trim and sexy figure that you want, there are countless options. You may have heard about exercising, getting your cardios right and dieting. You may have even tried all this methods. I bet you have not heard anything about

Intermittent fasting... right? Intermittent fasting is simply a way of changing or switching your diet patterns to make sure that you eat during different times in a day. It is also called the 5/2 Diet. This means that for 5 days you get to eat whatever you want and then for the next 2 days you cut down of the calories that you take in. The simple truth is that fasting is bad for you. But when done correctly, intermittent fasting can help you lose weight in the long run. Intermittent fasting makes you lose a lot of weight simply because you get to fast during certain parts of the week. This makes you stronger and healthier in the long run. Recent research has that many people who tried this diet have had their lives changed simply by the amount of fat they lost. According to Brad Pillon, the author of the popular Eat Stop Eat, he said that "In the fasted state, your body is set up to burn the calories that you stored while eating" so it is set up specifically for burning fat. How does it work? Intermittent fasting works simply by following a set dieting plan. First you eat normally for the first 5 days and then for the next 2 days you take in less than 600 calories. Simple and very easy to follow... So for example, if you start to implement this diet of Monday, then from Monday to Friday you get to eat all you like and then on Saturday and Sunday, you cut down on your calorie intake. How do I Start? • Firstly, all weight loss decisions starts with making a committed decision to stick to your plan. Yes even one such as this that involves you eating all you can and then cutting down for some days. You definitely need to be motivated to whatever plan you choose. • Also, weight loss is definitely easier when you eat whole, processed foods. Mind where you get your carbs from. Stick to fruits and vegetables instead of processed foods and you will be okay. A simple methodology of that you can apply immediately. You can eat breakfast on the first day and then the next meal that you take should be on the next day. Try varying the meal times to see what works. Do not despair and give up hope almost immediately. Weight loss is easy and simple to achieve. All you need is to make up your mind and you will be able to achieve it. Other benefits Include:

1. Changes the function of hormones, cells, and genes When you don't eat for a while, several things happen in your body. For example, your body changes hormone levels to make stored body fat more accessible and initiates important cellular repair processes.

Here are some of the changes that occur in your body during fasting:

Insulin levels. Blood levels of insulin drop significantly, which facilitates fat burning.

Human growth hormone (HGH) levels. The blood levels of human growth hormone (HGH) may increase dramatically. Higher levels of this hormone facilitate fat burning and muscle gain, and have numerous other benefits

Cellular repair. The body induces important cellular repair processes, such as removing waste material from cells.

Gene expression. There are beneficial changes in several genes and molecules related to longevity and protection against disease

Many of the benefits of intermittent fasting are related to these changes in hormones, the function of cells, and gene expression.

SUMMARY

When you fast, insulin levels drop and human growth hormone (HGH) increases. Your cells also initiate important cellular repair processes and change which genes they express.

2. Can help you lose weight and visceral fat

Many of those who try intermittent fasting are doing it to lose weight.

Generally speaking, intermittent fasting will make you eat fewer meals. Unless you compensate by eating much more during the other meals, you'll end up taking in fewer calories. Additionally, intermittent fasting enhances hormone function to facilitate weight loss. Lower insulin levels, higher HGH levels, and increased amounts of norepinephrine (noradrenaline) all increase the breakdown of body fat and facilitate its use for energy.

For this reason, short-term fasting actually increases your metabolic rate, helping you burn even more calories.

In other words, intermittent fasting works on both sides of the calorie equation. It boosts your metabolic rate (increases calories out) and reduces the amount of food you eat (reduces calories in).

According to a 2014 review of the scientific literature, intermittent fasting can cause weight loss of 3–8% over 3–24 weeks. This is a huge amount

The study participants also lost 4–7% of their waist circumference over 6–24 weeks, which indicates that they lost lots of visceral fat. Visceral fat is the harmful fat in the abdominal cavity that causes disease.

One 2011 review also showed that intermittent fasting caused less muscle loss than continuous calorie restriction.

However, a 2020 randomized trial looked at people who followed the 16/8 method. In this diet, you fast for 16 hours a day and have an 8-hour window to eat. The people who fasted didn't lose significantly more weight than the people who ate three meals a day. After testing a subset of the participants in person, the researchers also found that the people who fasted lost a significant amount of lean mass. This included lean muscle.

More studies are needed on the effect of fasting on muscle loss. All things considered, intermittent fasting has the potential to be an incredibly powerful weight loss tool.

SUMMARY

Intermittent fasting helps you eat fewer calories while boosting metabolism slightly. It's a very effective tool to lose weight and visceral fat.

3. Can reduce insulin resistance, lowering your risk for type 2 diabetes

Type 2 diabetes has become a very common diagnosis in recent decades.

Its main feature is high blood sugar levels in the context of insulin resistance. Anything that reduces insulin resistance should help lower blood sugar levels and protect against type 2 diabetes.

Interestingly, intermittent fasting has been shown to have major benefits for insulin resistance and to lead to an impressive reduction in blood sugar levels.

In human studies on intermittent fasting, fasting blood sugar has been reduced by 3–6% over the course of 8–12 weeks in people with prediabetes. Fasting insulin has been reduced by 20–31%.

One study in mice with diabetes also showed that intermittent fasting improved survival rates and protected against diabetic retinopathy. Diabetic retinopathy is a complication that can lead to blindness.

What this implies is that intermittent fasting may be highly protective for people who are at risk for developing type 2 diabetes.

However, there may be some differences between the sexes. One 2005 study in women showed that blood sugar management actually worsened after a 22-day long intermittent fasting protocol.

SUMMARY

Intermittent fasting can reduce insulin resistance and lower blood sugar levels, at least in men.

4. Can reduce oxidative stress and inflammation in the body

Oxidative stress is one of the steps toward aging and many chronic diseases. It involves unstable molecules called free radicals. Free radicals react with other important molecules, such as protein and DNA, and damage them.

Several studies show that intermittent fasting may enhance the body's resistance to oxidative stress.

Additionally, studies show that intermittent fasting can help fight inflammation, another key driver of many common diseases.

SUMMARY

Studies show that intermittent fasting can reduce oxidative damage and inflammation in the body. This should have benefits against aging and development of numerous diseases.

5. May be beneficial for heart health

Heart disease is currently the world's biggest killer.

It's known that various health markers (so-called "risk factors") are associated with either an increased or decreased risk of heart disease.

Intermittent fasting has been shown to improve numerous different risk factors, including:

- Blood sugar levels
- Blood pressure
- Blood triglycerides
- Total and ldl (bad) cholesterol

- Inflammatory markers

However, much of this is based on animal studies.
The effects of fasting on heart health need to be studied more in-depth in humans before recommendations can be made.

SUMMARY
Studies show that intermittent fasting can improve numerous risk factors for heart disease, such as blood pressure, cholesterol levels, triglycerides, and inflammatory markers.

6. Induces various cellular repair processes
When we fast, the cells in the body initiate a cellular "waste removal" process called autophagy. This involves the cells breaking down and metabolizing broken

and dysfunctional proteins that build up inside cells over time.

Increased autophagy may provide protection against several diseases, including cancer and neurodegenerative diseases such as Alzheimer's disease.

SUMMARY

Fasting triggers a metabolic pathway called autophagy, which removes waste material from cells.

7. May help prevent cancer

Cancer is characterized by uncontrolled growth of cells.

Fasting has been shown to have several beneficial effects on metabolism that may lead to reduced risk of cancer.

Promising evidence from animal studies indicates that intermittent fasting or diets that mimic fasting may help prevent cancer. Research in humans has led to similar findings, although more studies are needed.

There's also some evidence showing that fasting reduced various side effects of chemotherapy in humans.

SUMMARY

Intermittent fasting has been shown to help prevent cancer in animal studies and some human studies. Research in humans showed that it can help reduce side effects caused by chemotherapy.

8. Has benefits for your brain

What's good for the body is often good for the brain as well. Intermittent fasting improves various metabolic features known to be important for brain health.

Intermittent fasting helps reduce:

- Oxidative stress
- Inflammation
- Blood sugar levels
- Insulin resistance

Several studies in mice and rats have shown that intermittent fasting may increase the growth of new nerve cells, which should have benefits for brain function.

Fasting also increases levels of a brain hormone called brain-derived neurotrophic factor (BDNF). A BDNF deficiency has been implicated in depression and various other brain problems.

Animal studies have also shown that intermittent fasting protects against brain damage due to strokes.

SUMMARY

Intermittent fasting may have important benefits for brain health. It may increase growth of new neurons and protect the brain from damage.

9. May help prevent Alzheimer's disease

Alzheimer's disease is the world's most common neurodegenerative disease.

There's no cure currently available for Alzheimer's, so preventing it from showing up in the first place is critical.

Studies in rats and mice show that intermittent fasting may delay the onset of Alzheimer's or reduce its severity.

In a series of case reports, a lifestyle intervention that included daily short-term fasts was able to significantly improve Alzheimer's symptoms in 9 out of 10 people.

Animal studies also suggest that fasting may protect against other neurodegenerative diseases, including Parkinson's disease and Huntington's disease.

However, more research in humans is needed.

SUMMARY

Studies in animals suggest that intermittent fasting may be protective against neurodegenerative diseases such as Alzheimer's disease.

10. May extend your lifespan, helping you live longer

One of the most exciting applications of intermittent fasting may be its ability to extend lifespan.

Studies in rodents has shown that intermittent fasting extends lifespan in a similar way as continuous calorie restriction.

Intermittent fasting has also been shown to increase the lifespans of fruit flies.

In some of these studies, the effects were quite dramatic. In an older study, rats that were fasted every other day lived 83% longer than rats who weren't fasted.

In a 2017 study, mice that were fasted every other day saw their lifespans increase by around 13%

Daily fasting was also shown to improve the overall health of male mice. It helped delay the onset of conditions such as fatty liver disease and hepatocellular carcinoma, which are both common in aging mice.

Although this is far from being determined in humans, intermittent fasting has become very popular among the anti-aging crowd.

Given the known benefits for metabolism and all sorts of health markers, it makes sense that intermittent fasting could help you live a longer and healthier life.

SUMMARY

Intermittent fasting may help you live longer, according to studies in animals.

HOW TO START INTERMITTENT FASTING

Some people can flip a switch and jump right into intermittent fasting, but others need to modify their eating behaviors gradually. I count myself in that group! It took me some months to adopt intermittent fasting habits; I was addicted to food, stumbling to the pantry for breakfast each morning before I was even awake. It's ingrained in our psyche to eat a huge breakfast and snack throughout the day, so it may take time to acclimate to eating less. Maybe you start intermittent fasting Monday, Wednesday, Friday, or just on the weekend. Whatever works for you to get the ball rolling.

When talking to patients every day who practice commitment and discipline in their careers, finances, faith, and relationships, but food is the one obstacle they struggle to control. Intermittent fasting strips away the complexities and questions that surround most other popular weight loss and wellness strategies.

Without the mask of confusion, it's easy to identify exactly how to master intermittent fasting and achieve your goals.

Step 1: Cut Out Breakfast

The best and easiest way to begin intermittent fasting is to cut breakfast out of your routine. Your body works its own magic in the morning. Food only interrupts it. Cortisol hormones and adrenals surge in the morning to help you wake up, become alert, and generate energy. Why not take advantage of your body's natural rhythm to maximize the benefits of fasting?

Step 2: Find The Best Time To Workout

Many people make the mistake of thinking they can't workout while they're fasting, but the opposite is true. The morning is the best time for a vigorous workout! You're fresh and have hormonal optimization on your side.

Afternoon and evening workouts aren't always as effective as they could be; you're fatigued from the day, consumed with whatever new stressors landed in your lap at work, and are fighting the urge to slip off your shoes and unwind.

I was loyal to my afternoon workout routine for more than a decade, but switching to an early morning gym schedule has been a game-changer. If I don't workout first thing in the morning, I can practically see the sliding scale as I lose my opportunity throughout the day for a quality workout. Life gets busy, and the body gets drained!

Step 3: Relax. You Can Still Drink Your (Unsweetened) Coffee!

I know what you're about to ask with a hint of panic in your voice: "I can still drink coffee while I fast, right!?"

Yes! Luckily for coffee drinkers everywhere, our favorite morning ritual doesn't boost your blood sugar or disrupt your fast.

If you can't stomach the idea of black coffee, then yes, it's okay to add some creamer... but not too much! Keep in mind that your body will have to burn through the fat in the creamer before it can get back to burning your stored fat.

What about coffee drinkers who need to mask its bitterness with a sweetener? Zane warns against all-natural sweeteners, including cane sugar, honey, and agave. It's true that they're "natural" sugars, but they immediately send blood sugar and insulin levels surging. This in turn kicks your body out of its fasting period altogether.

If you need a hint of sweetness in your coffee, stick to a small dash of Stevia. Most artificial sugars are dangerous because they stimulate cravings and trick your digestive system into preparing for sugar that isn't coming. This is highly disruptive to the fat-burning process that fasting is meant to achieve.

Overall, the question of coffee boils down to your goals. If you're on a mission to lose 50 pounds, adding cream to your morning brew could slow your progress. But a sweetened cup of coffee is much better than a slice of cheesecake! It's all about balance.

Step 4. Diabetics, This Is For You, Too!

After Years of working regularly with diabetic clients who believe intermittent fasting poses too much of a risk.

But as he explains, "I don't know of a better way to control diabetes or reverse those symptoms than finding some way to introduce fasting."

Type 2 diabetes is a disease of elevated blood sugar, and intermittent fasting is an efficient way to lower and balance blood sugar levels through better eating strategies. In practice, fasting might just be the greatest tool my patients have to improve their glycemic control. As long as it's accomplished using a strategic, doctor-guided plan, diabetics may be able to use fasting to eliminate their reliance on medication and reduce the effects of diabetes.

Step 5: Use The Rhythms Of Fasting To Schedule Lunch And Dinner

You've heard enough; you're ready to dive head-first into the wonderful world of intermittent fasting. So when, exactly, can you eat?

The simplest approach nis skipping breakfast, (and) having coffee or tea. If your goal is weight loss, eat a low-carb lunch and dinner."

Your first meal of the day takes place after your fasting window ends, which means all of your eating occurs in a compressed window of about six to eight hours. That's give or take. Make it work with your schedule, If it's six hours, great. If it has to be nine one day, don't beat yourself up. That's the beauty of intermittent fasting: there's no right or wrong. It's one tool to improve your health in whatever way makes sense with your routine.

THE BOTTOM LINE

Intermittent fasting is a weight loss tool that works for many people, though it doesn't work for everyone. Some people believe it may not be as beneficial for women as for men. It's also not recommended for people who have or are prone to eating disorders. If you decide to try intermittent fasting, keep in mind that diet quality is crucial. It's not possible to binge on junk foods during the eating periods and expect to lose weight and boost your health.